Table of Contents

6

The Complete Quick and Easy Guides to

SCALP MICROPIGMENT ATION

In- Depth Information to Know Before Getting a Hair Tattoo and How to Feel Great About Yourself Again

Dr. JANE SCOTT

6

The Complete Quick and Easy Guides to

SCALP MICROPIGMENTATION

VOL. 2

In-Depth Information to Know Before Getting a Hair Tattoo and How to Feel Great About Yourself Again

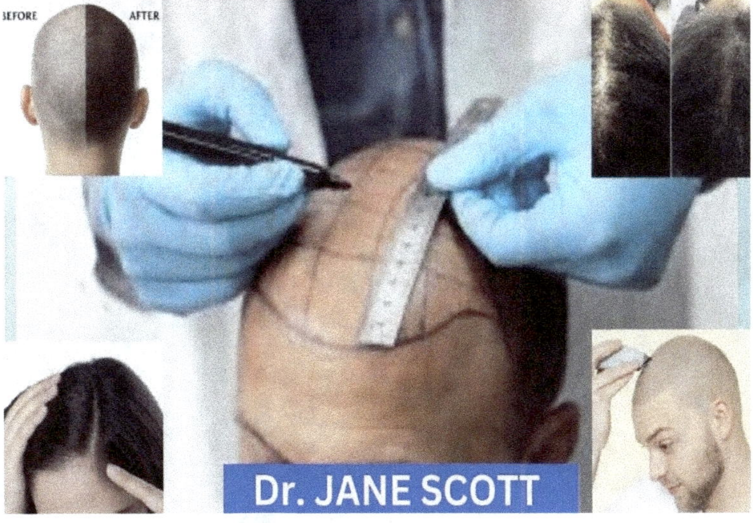

Dr. JANE SCOTT

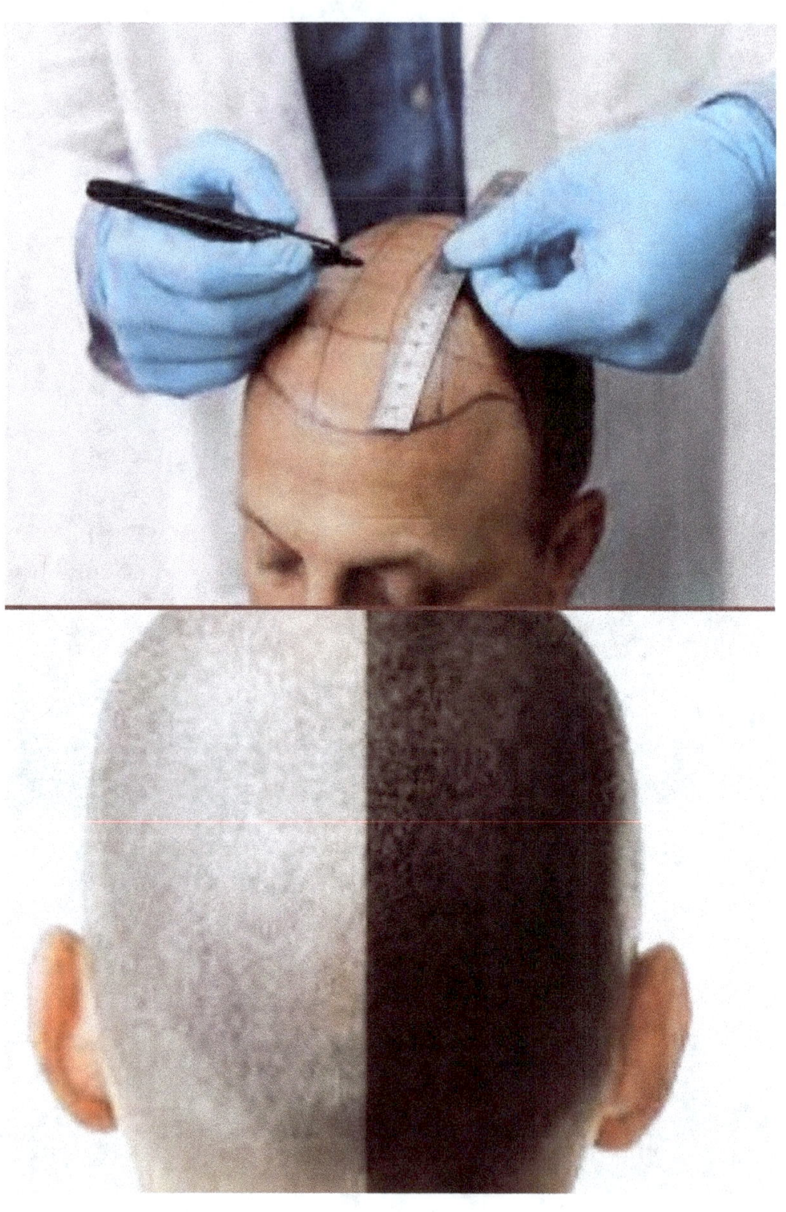

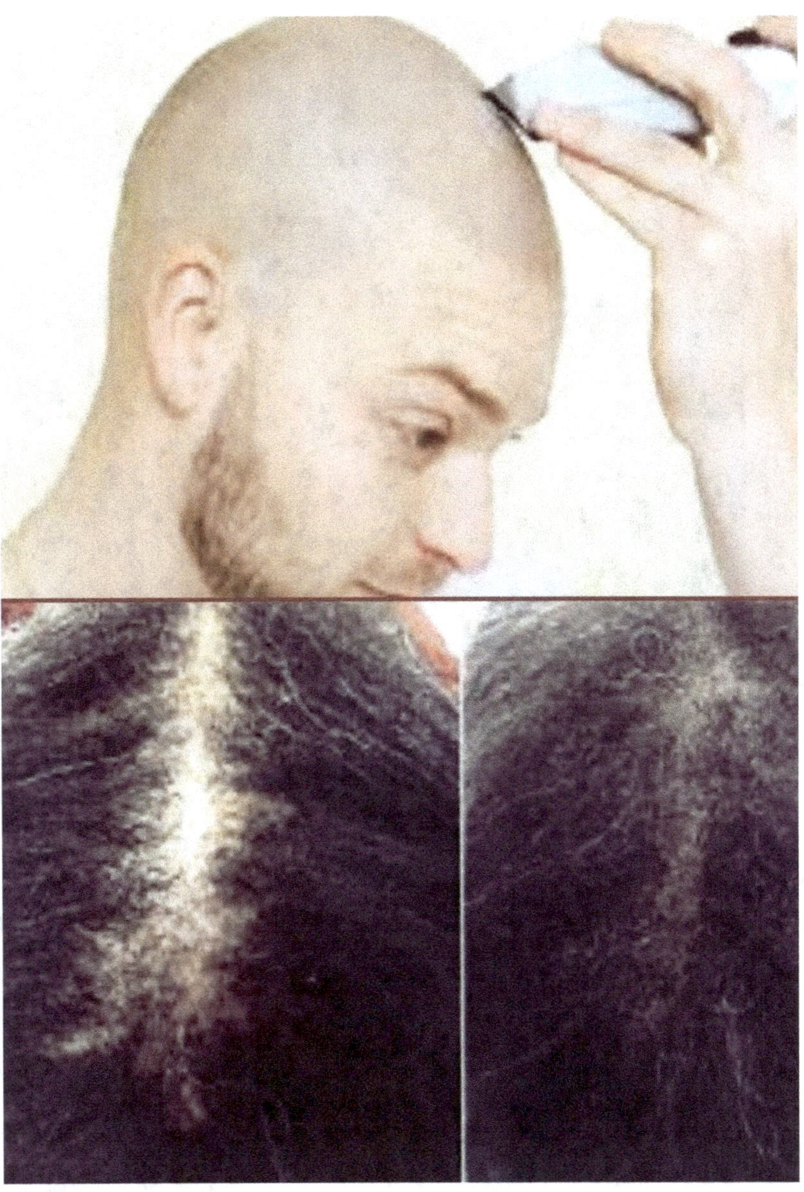

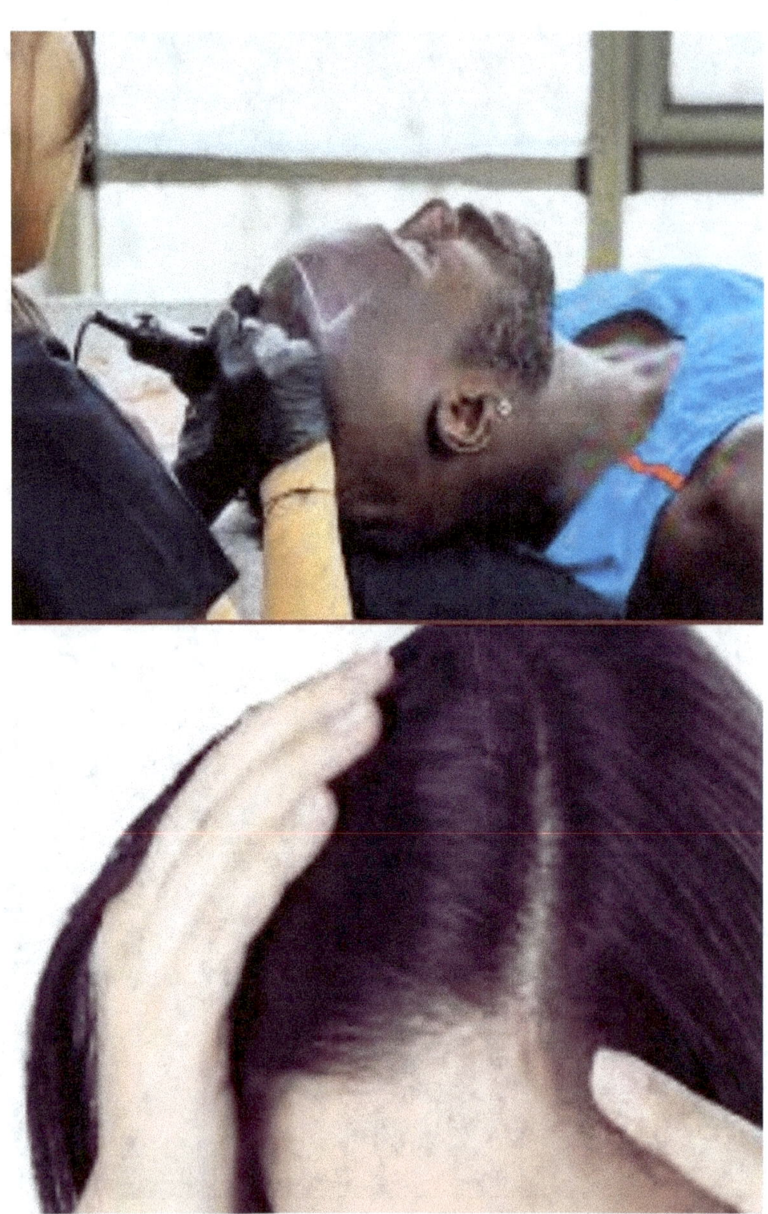

SMP STUDENT GUIDE

Scalp Micropigmentation (SMP) has emerged as a groundbreaking solution in the realm of cosmetic and aesthetic procedures, effectively addressing hair loss and thinning hair in a remarkable and innovative manner. This cutting-edge technique has gained significant popularity for its ability to create the illusion of a fuller head of hair by replicating the appearance of tiny hair follicles on the scalp. Whether due to genetics, medical conditions, or aging, hair loss can profoundly impact one's self-esteem and confidence. SMP offers a unique avenue to regain a sense of self-assurance and aesthetic satisfaction.

At its core, Scalp Micropigmentation is a non-invasive procedure involving the application of specialized pigments to the scalp using microfine needles. A skilled technician carefully deposits these pigments in a stippling pattern, meticulously mimicking the appearance of real hair follicles. This process results in the look of a closely shaved or buzzed hairstyle, providing the illusion of a full and dense head of hair. While SMP is often associated with treating male pattern baldness, it is equally effective for women experiencing hair thinning or partial hair loss.

One of the remarkable aspects of SMP is its versatility. It can be tailored to suit various degrees of hair loss, from minor thinning to more extensive balding. Additionally, SMP is not limited to head hair alone; it can also be used to address receding hairlines, thin eyebrows, and even camouflage scars resulting from hair transplant surgeries or accidents. The ability to customize SMP to an individual's unique needs is a testament to its adaptability and effectiveness.

Another key advantage of SMP is its low-maintenance nature. Unlike surgical hair restoration procedures, SMP does not require extensive downtime or follow-up procedures. The results are immediately noticeable, and the pigment's longevity ensures that clients enjoy their enhanced appearance for an extended period. Touch-up sessions may be needed over time to maintain the vibrancy and consistency of the pigment, but the overall upkeep is minimal compared to other hair restoration options.

As with any cosmetic procedure, thorough research and consultation with a certified SMP practitioner are essential steps for those considering the treatment. Understanding the process, potential outcomes, and post-procedure care is crucial in making an informed decision. With advancements in technology and the expertise of skilled practitioners, Scalp Micropigmentation offers a life-changing solution for individuals seeking to regain their confidence, improve their self-image, and embrace a renewed sense of pride in their appearance. Whether addressing hair loss head-on or enhancing specific features, SMP stands as an impressive testament to the fusion of artistry and science in modern aesthetics.

INTRODUCTIONS

WHAT IS SMP?

SMP, or scalp micropigmentation, entails the needle-based micropigmentation of pigment into the upper layers of the scalp. Little duplicate dots are created as a result of this process, each one resembling a unique human hair follicle. By carefully integrating these dots with any remaining real hair, it is possible to achieve the illusion of a completely styled head of hair. The effects of this intervention depend on three main factors: the skill and disposition of the technician, the clinical materials and techniques, and the particulars of the treatment.

HOW LONG HAS SCALP MICROPIGMENTATION BEEN AROUND?

Although it is still regarded as a relatively recent technique, records show that the first scalp microblading procedure occurred in the 1970s. Initially resembling a Õcalp tattoo, this technique used tattoo ink. Today's techniques, however, have changed dramatically, using warmer colors and patterns that produce results that look more natural. Interestingly, the process was not fully developed until 2002, and the first comprehensive treatment became available to the general public in 2006.

WHAT ABOUT 3D SCALP MICROPIGMENTATION?

This is a scam that is only used for advertising and to get people to call the company to get your business. A 3D Scalp Micropigmentation treatment is the only one of its kind. The color that is injected into the skin is flat and will stay flat until it fades.

Watch out for clinics that say they can do your SMP treatment in 3D just to get your business. Three dimensions are what 3D stands for: length, width, and depth. Point or snk does not have depth, of course.

But you wouldn't want a 3D dot on your head that gives it depth. There are 3D drawings and 3D tattoos. And so, there is no such thing as a 3D Scanning Micropigmentation Treatment. A good SMP clinic won't say they can do something that they can't, because they're just trying to get ahead of other clinics by making false claims.

• The middle segment is a short section that extends from the insertion of the erector pili muscle to the entrance of the sebaceous gland duct.

15

• The upper segment extends from the entrance of the sebaceous gland duct to the follicular orifice.

HAIRLOSS

WHAT IS HAIRLOSS?

The American Academy of Dermatology (AAD) notes that 80 million men and women in America have hereditary hair loss (alopecia). It can affect just the hair on your scalp or your entire body. Although alopecia is more prevalent in older adults, excessive hair loss can occur in children as well. It's normal to lose between 50 and 100 hairs a day. With about 100,000 hairs on your head, that small loss isn't noticeable. New hair normally replaces the lost hair, but this doesn't always happen. Hair loss can develop gradually over years or happen abruptly. Hair loss can be permanent or temporary. It's impossible to count the amount of hair lost on a given day. You may be losing more hair than is normal if you notice a large amount of hair in the drain after washing your hair or clumps of hair in your brush. You might also notice thinning patches of hair or baldness.

If your client notices that they are losing more hair than usual, they should discuss the problem with their doctor.

They can determine the underlying cause of hair loss and suggest appropriate treatment plans.

WHAT CAUSES HAIR LOSS?

The most common cause of hair loss is hereditary male- or female-pattern baldness. A family history of baldness may cause this type of hair loss. Certain sex hormones can trigger hereditary hair loss. It may begin as early as puberty. In some cases, hair loss may occur with a simple halt in the cycle of hair growth.

Major illnesses, surgeries, or traumatic events can trigger hair loss. However, the hair will usually start growing back without treatment.

HAIR LOSS CAUSES IN MEN

Throughout history, man has searched for the cause of hair loss. It is only in recent years, with greater knowledge of genetics and the chemistry of sexual hormones, that we have begun to understand the causes. One thing that we do know for certain: no matter what we eat, what our lifestyles may be, or what kind of vitamins we take, we never grow more hair follicles than we were born with.

Gene

Hormones

Age

The average Caucasian is born with 100,000 hairs, the average Asian with 80,000 hairs, and the average African with 60,000 hairs. The character and the thickness of each hair shaft reflect the ability of that hair to cover the scalp.

Fine hair covers less than coarse hair. Curly hair covers better than straight hair (e.g., African hair, with its kinky character, covers well, especially when the hair is coarser.) Straight hair layers well, so most people with straight hair take advantage of styling to maximize the coverage that straight hair brings.

The most common type of baldness is called Male Pattern Baldness, or, more scientifically, Androgenetic Alopecia. In Androgenetic Alopecia, hair follicles that are producing healthy, terminal hairs begin to produce thinner, shorter, more brittle hairs with weaker shafts (this process is called Miniaturization, and the hairs involved are called Miniaturized hairs).

Eventually, these follicles produce only fine, almost invisible, short, vellus-like hairs, or they may die out altogether. The dying process of a hair from Androgentic Alopecia is called Apotosis, and the timing of this process is ingrained in the genetics of balding. It is regional, varying in different parts of the scalp. The patterns of male pattern balding reflect the apoptosis (life cycle) of the hair, and the areas that lose their hair eventually undergo apoptosis. Fortunately, the hair around the back and sides of the head seems to be immune from Apoptosis, and these hairs live if most humans who, when they die, will still have this rim of hair around the side and back of the head, even in the baldest of men.

Androgenetic hair loss is caused by the effects of male hormones on genetically susceptible hair follicles. It is related to three interdependent factors:

Overall thinning

Bald spots

Handfuls of hair

Full loss

HAIR LOSS IN WOMEN

Hair loss is common for women, too There are numerous reasons why women might experience hair loss. Anything from medical conditions to hormonal changes to stress may be the culprit. It's not always easy tracing the root cause, but here are some of the possibilities and what you can do.

SIGNS OF HAIR LOSS

Hair loss may present in different ways depending on the cause. You may notice sudden hair loss or a gradual thinning over time. It may be helpful to keep a diary to track any changes you notice or symptoms you experience, and to look for patterns.

Certain signs include:

Gradual thinning on the top of the head is the most common type of hair loss. It affects both men and women. While men tend to see a receding hairline, women generally notice that their part broadens.

They may be circular or patchy. They may resemble coins in size and usually appear on the scalp. Your skin may even feel itchy or painful immediately before the hair falls out. You may experience very sudden hair loss, particularly after emotional or physical trauma. The hair may come out quickly while you're washing or combing it, leading to overall thinning. In some medical situations, particularly with medical treatments like chemotherapy, you may notice hair loss suddenly and all over your body at once.

Men are not the only people who suffer from hair loss. While male pattern baldness is a more common and accepted condition, many practitioners perform SMP for women just as often as their male clients.

Androgenetic alopecia is female-pattern baldness or hair loss caused by genetics, or family history. It's the leading cause of hair loss in women and generally begins between the ages of 12 to 40 years old. While men tend to notice balding as a receding hairline and specific bald spots, women's hair loss appears more as overall thinning.

Alopecia areata is patchy hair loss that happens suddenly on the head or body. It typically begins with one or more round bald patches that may or may not overlap. Cicatricial alopecia is a group of conditions that causes irreversible hair loss through scarring. Hair falls out and the follicle is replaced with scar tissue. Traumatic alopecia's cause hair to fall out because of hair styling practices. The hair shaft may break after using hot combs, blow dryers, straighteners, or certain chemicals to dye or straighten hair.

There are several reasons why women could begin losing their hair. Alopecia is an autoimmune condition that can cause hair loss all over the body, and often presents with hair falling out in chunks, leaving the patient with large bald spots all over his or her head.

Women are often under an immense amount of social pressure to look great, and one way many choose to accomplish this is to restrictively diet to lose those extra pounds. Unfortunately, if a diet doesn't provide the body with the nutrients it needs, one could end up shedding hair alongside weight. Hair loss is wrapped up in genetics, and just like men, certain women may be predisposed. Next, we'll look at major types of hair loss and causes.

TYPES OF ALOPECIA

Alopecia simply means "hair loss." It's not contagious or attributed to nerves. There are a variety of types caused by anything from genetics to hair care practices or anything that triggers the immune system to attack hair follicles. To understand the different types of hair loss in women, and

21

their management, it is helpful to divide the patterns into three broad categories:

LOCALIZED HAIR LOSS

Localized hair loss may be sub-divided into scarring and non-scarring types. Alopecia Areata is a genetic, auto-immune disease that typifies the non-scarring type. It manifests itself with the sudden onset of round patches of hair loss associated with normal skin and can be treated with local injections of Cortico steroids. Scarring Alopecia can be caused by a variety of medical or dermatologic conditions such as Lupus and Lichen Planus, or local radiation therapy. Baldness from injuries, or from local medical problems that have been cured, are usually amenable to hair transplantation. Localized hair loss that occurs around the hairline after face-lift surgery may be permanent as can Traction Alopecia, the hair loss that occurs with constant tugging on the hair. Both conditions can be treated with hair transplantation.

PATTERNED HAIR LOSS

Women with this type of hair loss have a pattern but this pattern differs from the classic male patterns shown in the Norwood Scale for men's hair loss. There are two types of patterns seen in women. One pattern is like the 'A' variants where the male loses only frontal hair which can progress to the swirl. This frontal pattern is often stronger in the front like what we observe in men. In other words, they have thinning in front progressively to the top of their scalp with little hair loss in the permanent zone around the sides and in the back.

The second type of patterned female hair loss reflects thinning behind the hairline from the front to the vertex (swirl area) and this thinning is often uniform and progressive. This second type is more common than the first type discussed above. Thus, the balding process occurs in a characteristic "pattern" rather than generalized thinning throughout the scalp. Depending upon the degree of hair loss and its distribution, women with patterned hair loss may be excellent candidates for surgical restoration provided that the donor hair (around the sides and back of the head) remain normal without significant miniaturization.

DIFFUSE HAIR LOSS

A third category of hair loss in women is a generalized thinning that affects all parts of the scalp. This is the most common type of hair loss seen in females. In this situation, much of the hair remains, but the thickness of the hair shaft is smaller than normal hair. The medical term for this type of thinning is "Diffuse Un-patterned Alopecia". These women have thinning that involves the donor area so that women with this type of hair loss are generally not good candidates for surgery.

Because diffuse hair loss can be caused by a variety of conditions other than "hereditary balding" women who are losing their hair should be evaluated by a physician who is experienced with these problems. Most important, they should know when a medical evaluation is appropriate and whether medical or surgical treatments will offer the greatest benefit.

WHY SMP FOR WOMEN IS AN IMPORTANT PROCEDURE

It may seem like there are few options for women who are losing their hair. After all, not every girl can pull off a short hairstyle. The situation is not so hopeless, however. Even if wigs, special shampoos, and surgeries haven't done the job, Scalp Micropigmentation isn't short hair specific! Patients can choose how to fill out their visible scalp.

ASSESSING HAIR LOSS

The first step in assessing the extent of your client's hair loss is to compare their current hairline with a photograph taken a few years ago. This will give you an approximate idea of the amount and rate of hair loss. A common issue for many men is not knowing the extent of hair loss in the crown area. To accurately assess hair loss in this area, take a picture of the back of the head in good lighting or with a flash.

Understanding the hair loss patterns of your client's father, grandfather, and brothers can help predict what might happen to your client. While they may not follow the same patterns, it provides a reasonable estimate of potential hair loss.

A thorough history and examination of the scalp can reveal the extent and trend of the hair loss process. Using a Hair Densitometer, a magnifying device invented by Dr. William Rassman, and a hair check instrument that measures hair bulk, you can determine the actual degree of hair loss in various scalp areas. This establishes a baseline to grade hair loss over time. If you treat the hair loss with a drug like Minoxidil, a repeat examination in 6-12 months can show the treatment's effectiveness.

Careful assessment of the hair loss process is critical for accurately predicting the rate and extent of hair loss. We have seen young men without any visible hair loss convinced they are losing hair. By measuring hair bulk in different areas with the hair check instrument, we can validate or reject this belief, as the eye cannot detect a loss of up to 30% or more of the hair in any area.

The scientific way to assess the degree of baldness is to compare your client's pattern with standard patterns. The Regular Type is characterized by hair loss beginning in two areas (the hairline and crown) that gradually merge. The less common Type "A" pattern is characterized by "front-to-back" hair loss. In men, 99% of hair loss is genetic, and hair loss that is not genetic usually does not conform to these patterns.

MALE HAIR LOSS MEASUREMENT

In 1975, Dr. O'Tar Norwood developed a classification of male pattern hair loss that is widely used today. He divided androgenetic hair loss in men into two common patterns:

Some women also lose hair according to the pattern described by Norwood, but more commonly have a diffuse thinning process (thinning all over), rather than patterned variety. Pattern balding does occur in women, but when they do, they do not develop the patterns described by Norwood, but rather patterns described by Hamilton. The Norwood patterns shown below do not progress from 2 to 7. The hairs that are lost in these male patterns form a gradual process. In other words, if your father has a Class 7 pattern, he developed it most probably before the age of 30, often never going though the other patterns shown below.

Hair loss always progresses over the years, although the rate can vary dramatically from person to person, and the rate of loss can vary significantly.

For example, a man may lose hair rapidly in his early 40s and then stabilize for many years, not showing a significant amount of additional hair loss until his 60s. People who become extensively bald usually show most of their hair loss in their 20s (but not always). It is the doctor's job to help you slow this progression down with the use of medications that often work well.

In general, the pattern of one's hair loss follows the specific type first presented. On a thorough examination by a good doctor, the bulk measurements, regardless of what can be seen with the naked eye, will show loss of bulk in the Class 5 pattern despite the reality that what you see may just be a Class 3 pattern. A Class 3 pattern may become a Class 4 and then a Class 5 pattern, but again, the bulk measurements will mostly show some early hair loss in the entire Class 5 pattern, regardless of what you see. Rarely, a Class 2 may thin diffusely and directly evolve into a Class 6 or 7 pattern.

The patterns you see in your older relatives may become your pattern since heredity plays an important role in androgenetic baldness. It is important to know the age at which the family member reached a specific pattern. For example, if your clients father was totally bald but lost all his hair in his 20s, and your client is 35 with only a Class 4 pattern, his extensive hair loss pattern has little relevance to predicting your clients future hair loss.

TYPE 1

In this stage, hair loss is mild. Most women may have difficulty noticing that hair loss has occurred, as the frontal hairline remains relatively unaffected. Hair loss may occur on the top and front of the scalp.

Such hair loss may be noticeable when the hair is parted down the center of the scalp, as more and more scalp will become visible over time.

TYPE 2

This type of hair loss is considered moderate. In this stage, women may notice each of the following:

Thinning, shedding, general decrease in volume, and a center part that continues to widen over time. Depending on the severity, a hair transplant procedure may be a viable option for women who exhibit a Type 2 classification.

TYPE 3

This is the final and most extreme classification of female hair loss. In this stage, hair is so thin that it has difficulty camouflaging the scalp, rendering it visible to the naked eye. This may be worsened by several factors, including hair miniaturization, progressive thinning, and extensive loss.

FEMALE HAIR LOSS MEASUREMENT

The Ludwig scale is the generally accepted standard when describing and measuring the extent of female hair loss and uses 3 different classifications.

HAIRLINE TYPES

Reconstruction of a natural hairline and crown is the most requested service from patrons seeking relief from hair loss. Four sessions are normally completed to ensure the scalp has a healthy gradient, and a textured look that rivals the best artisans. A natural hairline is achieved by establishing a staggered hairline, which creates an implied line across the forehead. Once the perfect hair line is achieved based on symmetry, facial anatomy, and texture the crown of the scalp can be filled in to match native follicles. Natural hairlines are popular because the average person cannot tell your client has had anything done, and it is the closest match to their old hairline they you used to have prior to hair loss.

• Soft Hairline

Soft hairlines are for men and women who request a natural blending effect which is staggered with an implied line and no impressions at the temple areas. Natural hairlines are often done in very light passes to ensure the skin maintains a soft look by the end of the fourth session. Peppering is done at the fourth session to bring some pops of naturalism to the scalp, but the overall purpose of this look is to recreate the shaved follicle look to the front of the scalp. Soft hairlines are a client preference, and the outline placement will be determined based on facial symmetry, bone structure, and a rested or smiling state.

• Hard Hairline

Hard hairlines are for men and women who want a sharp barbered edge up with pointed edges at the temple areas. Normally hard hairlines can still be softened by staggering a few impressions outside of the hairline, yet still maintain a true line. Hard lines are requested by people who are used to going to the barber on the regular and wish to maintain a crisp outline at the front of the scalp. Hard lines can also be

29

altered into soft lines in the future if there is room left at the temple to bring the hairline down. Hard lines are a client preference, and the outline placement will be determined based on facial symmetry, bone structure, and a rested and smiling state.

• Hybrid Hairline

Hybrid hairlines are for men and women who want a slightly receded hairline which is very close to their natural hairline. Often the temple areas are rounded with minimal impressions. Hybrid hairlines are often requested when the client does not want to change their temple area but does want to bring their hairline down one to two inches. These kinds of hairlines are the most natural as they blend in effortlessly with the native follicles, but the temple area remains consistently with the current state of their hair loss. Normally this is reserved for those who want to do minimal work and wish to create a soft polished hairline. Placement will be determined based on facial symmetry, bone structure, and a rested or smiling state.

Restoration of the Original Hairline Faded, Soft and Broken

Defined but Receded

Broken and Jagged

Super Sharp and Defined

Aggressive Angles

30

Straight and Angular

Natural

Curving down of the hairline on the sides of the hairline

Lateral humps

Widow's peak

Long Hair

Density treatments are often used to rectify thinning for patrons with long hair. Normally technicians will implement three to five passes per session to stain the skin. The purpose of density for long hair treatments is normally to fill in the hairline, and temple areas. Long hair is heavy and often puts strain on the hairline which eventually breaks or becomes very weak and thin. On average density treatments are done along the hair line, or part line to bring color and thickness back to the area. Each session will reveal a darker hue to the scalp and ensure the hairline is properly placed back in its rightful position.

Curly Hair

Density treatments can be used for curly hair patterns. Often curls can leave bald spots that are very noticeable based on the direction of hair growth. The curl type can determine the density amount used based on the color, thickness, and wave pattern. Often a clean fade is used on the sides to establish a barber line up, and blended temple points

GUIDELINES TO CONSIDER

Things to Consider when creating a hairline:

Men with darker skin are better at pulling off super-sharp styles, straight hairlines, and aggressive angles. Faded hairlines can be less effective depending on skin color. They do not work on dark skin men. The requirement for minuscule dot size combined with a smaller variation in color between the pigment and the skin, usually results in the pigments fading very quickly or being less noticeable than desired from the moment they are applied.

The other optional alternations that should be considered when designing a female hairline, based on the shape and position of the other components of the face, are:

WHAT ARE THE DIFFERENT TYPES OF HAIRLINES FOR WOMEN AND MEN?

Hairlines are defined in men and women by several characteristics, such as shape and height. Every person's hairline is different and distinctive, but typically falls within one of several categories. Hairlines also change with age. If you have a hairline you don't like, you may be able to alter it. We'll go over the most common types of hairlines in men and women and discuss options for changing a hairline you're not happy with.

WHAT ARE THE DIFFERENT HAIRLINE TYPES FOR WOMEN?

Hairlines are affected by multiple factors, including genetics, hormones, age, and lifestyle habits. Just about any hairline can be styled to look attractive.

Hairline Types in Women Include

1. LOW HAIRLINE

Hairlines that sit relatively close to the eyebrows are considered low. Women with low hairlines give the appearance of having narrow, or short foreheads. Since hairlines in both men and women may recede with age, starting out with a low hairline could be an advantage.

2. HIGH HAIRLINE

If your hairline begins high up on the crown of your head, you have a high hairline. High hairlines are often the result of genetics but can also be caused by hair loss.

3. MIDDLE HAIRLINE

A middle hairline is also referred to as an average, or normal, hairline. This type of hairline sits in the middle of the forehead. While there's no actual data indicating the most common type of hairline in women, midline hairlines seem to be the most customary kind.

4. WIDOW'S PEAK

If your hairline has a distinctive V-shape, you have a widow's peak. This distinctive hairline may be inherited. It may also be the result of several rare genetic disorders, such as frontonasal dysplasia. Widow's peaks may become more prominent or less prominent with age.

lifestyle habits

hormones

genetics

stress

5. TRIANGULAR HAIRLINE

A triangular hairline has the opposite look of a widow's peak. It can also take on the appearance of a slightly off-center triangle, with the upwards point occurring on one side of the hairline. In some instances, a triangular hairline may be caused by temporal triangular alopecia, a condition also referred to as congenital triangular alopecia.

6. UNEVEN HAIRLINE

Lack of symmetry is common in hairlines. You may find that one side of your hairline is slightly higher than the other. You may also have a hairline that zig zags slightly, or significantly. Uneven hairlines can be the result of genetics. They can also be caused by hair styling practices, such as pulling or tugging the hair too tightly over time. A hairline can also become uneven if your hair starts to recede.

7. BELL-SHAPED

Rounded, oval, or bell-shaped hairlines are typically symmetrical. They may make the forehead appear long in shape. Bell-shaped hairlines have a curved look, with no uneven lines.

8. STRAIGHT-LINED

If your hairline is straight across your forehead, it's considered straight-lined, or rectangular in shape. This type of hairline is sometimes referred to as a juvenile hairline.

9. RECEDING HAIRLINE OR M-SHAPE

Receding hairlines in women are less common than they are in men. However, they're far from rare, and can be caused by: Receding hairlines in women differ from female pattern baldness (androgenic alopecia). If you have a receding hairline, your hair may stop growing at one or both temples, giving you an "M" shape. Your hairline may also recede straight back horizontally, exposing more of your entire forehead. Lifestyle habits, like wearing too-tight hairstyles every day for years, can cause a hairline to recede. This phenomenon may be temporary or permanent and is known as traction alopecia.

If your hair is treated regularly with chemicals, traction alopecia may be more likely to occur. Receding hairlines can also be related to the hormonal changes associated with menopause. Some women may notice that their hairlines have receded slightly at the temples after pregnancy. This type of hair loss is often temporary.

WHAT ARE THE DIFFERENT HAIRLINE TYPES FOR MEN?

Men can have any of the hairline shapes that woman do. The male hairline, however, can change much more dramatically over time.

Some Of the Most Common Hairline Types in Men Include

1. LOW HAIRLINE

Low hairlines in males may be most common in boys and young men, who have not yet started to experience any hair loss. When a low hairline is straight across, it's referred to as a juvenile hairline. As with women, a low hairline is one that starts closer to the eyebrows than the average hairline does. It gives the appearance of having a narrow forehead.

2. MIDDLE HAIRLINE

Men who have middle, or average hairlines have a proportionate look to their foreheads. This type of hairline is common in men, during their teens and twenties. A middle hairline may sometimes be uneven, or asymmetrical. It may also appear straight or rounded.

3. RECEDING HAIRLINE (MALE PATTERN BALDNESS)

Male pattern baldness is a hereditary trait, caused by the interplay between hair follicles and hormones, such as testosterone. This condition is also referred to as androgenetic alopecia.

Males may start to notice their hairlines begin to recede at any point after puberty. Receding hairlines can take on the appearance of high hairlines that continue to show more scalp as they recede. Receding hairlines in men can also cause a deep "M" shape, if the hair recedes dramatically at the temples.

4. COWLICK

Cowlicks are swirls of hair that grow in a direction other than their surrounding hairs. Cowlicks may occur anywhere on the scalp, but are often found at the crown, or hairline. Cowlicks know no gender and can occur in males and females. They are more commonly seen in men who have short hair, and few styling options for taming them.

HAIRLINE DESIGN

Establishing the midline to have a relatively balanced hairline Defining the proportions of the face based on the rule of thirds

Adjusting the front and corners accordingly

Adding micro-irregularities as a natural hairline always has it

Defining the priorities and budgeting the hair density in different areas strategically

Hairline design is one of the key elements of a hair restoration procedure. In most cases, knowing how to create a natural looking hairline is essential for SMP artists.

MALE HAIRLINE DESIGN

A good-looking face is often also considered to be a proportional face. We can see a special proportion in the face of most good-looking men and women. What we want to achieve with most patients is a face that is divided proportionately in three sections.

The distance between the tip of the nose to the bottom of the chin should be about the same as the hairline to the point between the eyebrows. This happens to fall to 7-8cm in most men. The creation of a hairline at the midline position of the forehead is what restores the proportions of the face in a good-looking man. A successful hairline design involves many steps including:

FEMALE HAIRLINE DESIGN

In comparison to a male hairline, women generally have the corners of their frontal hairline flat or lowered. This still falls into the category of proportional faces following the rule of thirds for vertical proportions at the middle. However, on the sides, the horizontal proportions should be considered, and the corners will be closer in a typical female hairline. Some women may have lateral humps that lower the hairline on both sides of the midline that falls into the definition of a feminine hairline. The most important alteration that should be followed for a female hairline is the lack of hairline recession on the sides (corners) of the frontal hairline.

Curving down of the hairline on the sides of the hairline

Lateral humps

Widow's peak

Clients in their 40's or older might want to choose a slightly more receded, age-appropriate look. Start with your original hairline position and factor in some widow's peaks and higher overall position.

Those with a naturally high hairline might want to bring their new hairline a little lower than its original position. This is perfectly acceptable however proceed with caution. Moderation is key. The other optional alternations that should be considered when designing a female hairline, based on the shape and position of the other components of the face, are:

SCALP MICROPIGMENTATION HAIRLINES

There are several factors that determine the success of your scalp micropigmentation treatment. Although some people prefer a 'statement' look, particularly younger clients, or those of Asian or African American descent, for most people the aim is a high level of realism. To create an illusion of hair that is convincing enough for your new look to never be questioned.

The most significant factor that determines the level of realism, is the position, shape, and design of your frontal hairline. This is because the hairline is the first thing you see when you look in the mirror, and the first thing other people see when they look at your 'hair'. It is important to realize that the human gaze is naturally drawn to straight lines. If you have an ultra-straight hairline, you're much more likely to be called out.

THE POSITION OF THE HAIRLINE

This should be a simple decision for most clients, but one that so many people get wrong. The best advice I can offer is to start with the position of your ORIGINAL hairline, before you started to lose your hair. It may help to refer to some old photos of your client.

A couple of exceptions:

THE SHAPE OF THE HAIRLINE

Real simple one this. In most cases I would recommend that you start with the shape of your ORIGINAL hairline and go with that. If you want to adjust, ensure they are only minor tweaks.

Remember you cannot change the shape of the face, and a hairline that is significantly different from the original is likely to draw unwanted attention. Straight hairlines are spotted a mile away, so only go for the Jamie Foxx look if you don't mind getting called out.

A nice, rounded hairline that works with the shape of the head is what you should be looking to achieve. Add widows' peaks, give a slight point at the center, or go for something more randomly shaped, but stay away from straight hairlines if you want your client to remain inconspicuous. Several American providers offer defined hairlines, but as natural looking hairlines have gotten more and more realistic, the defined look has fallen out of favor and tends to be the reserve of less-experienced technicians now, so it really shouldn't be chosen unless you're sure it's what you really want. Many people are now lasering off their old hairlines and opting for a more natural look.

THE STYLE OF THE HAIRLINE

This is the clincher. If you've followed my advice about the position and shape of your hairline, you're nearly there. Now make sure the finish of your hairline, the most important part, is executed professionally by an experienced technician. This part takes a certain degree of skill.

THE BROKEN OR JAGGED HAIRLINE

A broken hairline requires the scattering of random pigment deposits below the actual hairline, to simulate the natural distribution of real hair. The reason why broken hairlines are so popular is because they mimic the appearance of a natural hair pattern. Very few people have a naturally defined hairline, at least not without the help of a barber, so broken hairlines are best for recreating a person's original appearance.

Faded hairlines are not suitable for everyone. They do not work well on darker skin, or on clients that require lighter pigments. In both cases, the 'fade' tends to get lost and results in a more defined look than was intended. There is little the technician can do to avoid this. The best candidates have light skin with medium to dark hair, or medium skin with dark hair.

Even when the candidate is 'ideal', it takes a considerable level of skill to create this look. The technique is beyond the capability of the average scalp micropigmentation technician; therefore, it is essential that the right technician is sought, and evidence of their results is acquired prior to any commitment being made.

A jagged hairline takes the concept a step further, by breaking up the hairline more aggressively to remove any linear aspect to its appearance. Hairlines like these can work exceptionally well for some clients, and ultimately achieve the same goal as a broken hairline.

LIGHTWEIGHT HAIRLINES

A lightweight hairline, sometimes referred to as 'faded' 'feathered' or 'gradient', is applied with an extremely light touch with no 'line' whatsoever, to completely remove any boundary to the hairline, thus avoiding unwanted attention.

When executed correctly, lightweight hairlines push the boundaries of realism to new levels. Another lightweight hairline in a slightly different style.

If a lightweight hairline is what you want, there are two important considerations that you must consider:

THE 'EDGE-UP' HAIRLINE

Often combined with a defined hairline shape, an edge-up hairline is often referred to as a 'hard line' and involves no deviation from the intended hairline position. No pigments are scattered, and no attempt is made to break the hairline up. These hairlines are still popular among younger clients, particularly African American and Asian clients, however a natural appearance is not usually achieved. The style is best suited to those who want a 'statement' to look and aren't concerned about being called out.

Also, a word of caution. Nothing but edge-up hairlines in a technician's portfolio is often a sign of limited experience, or a sub-standard skill level.

DEFINED HAIRLINES

Defined hairlines are simpler to create than ultra realistic hairlines, and frankly, require less talent to produce. Don't be put off at all if a technician has hairlines like these in their portfolio but be mindful that they should be able to create a mix of hairlines, including the latest broken, jagged, and lightweight examples shown above. Defined hairlines are particularly popular and suitable for clients with darker skin, like this African American client above. Many of the terminologies like 'broken hairline', 'feathered hairline' and 'edge up' have become industry-standard terms.

A skilled scalp micropigmentation technician should be able to replicate any hairline style you desire, whether you want a totally natural appearance or a braver style.

COLOR THEORY & PIGMENTS

COLOR THEORY

THE COLOR WHEEL
The color wheel is a visual representation of colors arranged by their color values. Understanding the color wheel provides artists with important fundamental knowledge for proper pigment selection and color correction. The color wheel shows the relationships between primary colors, secondary colors and tertiary colors.

PRIMARY COLORS: RED / YELLOW / BLUE
They are considered primary colors because they cannot be made by mixing other colors together. These three colors are the base for every other color on the color wheel which is why they are considered primary.

SECONDARY COLORS: PURPLE / GREEN / ORANGE

When you mix primary colors together you get secondary colors. On the color wheel, they are located between the primary colors.

WARM COLORS: red, orange, and yellow

COOL COLORS: green, blue, and purple.

NEUTRAL COLORS: black, gray, white and brown.

There are three types of colors:

warm, cool, and neutral colors.

TYPES OF COLORS

BROWN

Mix 3 primary colors together to get brown: Yellow + Red + Blue.

Mix a primary color with a secondary color at the opposite spectrum of the color wheel to get brown:

Yellow + Purple Blue + Orange Red + Green

Brown is a tertiary color. There are 2 ways to achieve brown. In a perfect world, our brown color should have an equal component of each of the primary colors. Meaning a perfect brown would have an equal amount of each primary colors.

This information will become more important when we discuss color corrections (in a different section).

SKIN TONES

Exposure to the elements Medication

Sickness or disease

Smoking

Diet

Ingesting alcohol

Pregnancy

Understanding skin tones and undertones is important for finding the right color for your client and preventing residual color. Skin tone and undertone are two different things. Skin tone is your skin color. It's determined by the amount of skin pigment (melanin) in the uppermost layer of the skin. Undertone is the hue from underneath the surface of your skin. Skin tone can change overtime however undertone does not.

There are different ways to classify skin tone. You can classify skin type by using descriptions ranging from ivory to ebony or you can use a numerical scientific skin type classification commonly known as the Fitzpatrick Scale.

46

Overtone is the color that we see on the surface of the skin. It can be influenced by:

Hemoglobin - red; shows up as a blue undertone

Carotene – yellow

Melanin - brownish-black

In addition to skin tones, understanding the different undertones will allow you to know which pigments to choose for your clients and which pigments to avoid to prevent residual color. Undertones, unlike skin tones, never change and they are based on your skin's underlying hue. There are 3 major undertones: warm, cool and neutral.

Undertone is the underlying quality of the skin, and is a combination of 3 pigments: If your client's undertone is warm, you should avoid pigments with too much warmth. You should typically choose a pigment color that is slightly more cool neutral. This will prevent your client's brows from fading to red. If your client's undertone is cool, you should avoid pigments that are too cool. You should typically choose a pigment that is slightly more warm- neutral. This will prevent your client's brows from fading to grey. For neutral undertones, you should avoid choosing pigments that are both too warm or cool.

UNDERTONES

if gold suits better skin undertone is generally warm

if silver suits better skin undertone is generally warm

IDENTIFYING UNDERTONES

Hair color – A key example in deciding the undertones of your client is to look at the client's hair color. If it is natural decide if you see warm, cold, or neutral tones present. If the client colors their hair, determine what tones are in the hair colorant and if the tones suit the client. If a client has warm undertones in her hair, then she will need a warm based pigment selection and vice versa, If the client has cool undertones, then a cool based pigment.

In addition, hair is classified by undertone or chroma; here are some typical classifications:

R – Red

N – Neutral

G – Gold

A – Ash

V – Violet

JEWELLERY – DOES YOUR CLIENT WEAR JEWELLERY?

If so, is it silver, rose gold or gold? Does it suit them? Do they prefer to wear gold or silver? Or can they wear both? If the client wears and suits silver, then they generally are cold undertones. If they wear gold, then they will generally have warm undertones in their skin. If the client can wear both gold and silver, then they have neutral skin undertones.

PAPER TEST

It is a good idea to have two matte pieces of gold and silver card kept in the salon. When undergoing the skin tone analysis, you can hold up both colors of card one at a time, then both together at the side of the clients face and determine which color they will suit.

VEIN TEST

You can look at the client's veins on their wrist in natural daylight also as a way of determining the clients skin undertones. If a client has veins that look either blue or purple, then they are likely to have cool undertones. If the client's veins appear to look green or greeny blue, then the client generally will have warm undertones. If you can't tell what color the client's veins are then they generally will have neutral skin undertones.

The Fitzpatrick scale is a numerical, scientific system to classify skin color. This system is based on the amount of pigment in your skin and your skin's reaction to sun exposure. When choosing a pigment color for your client, it is important to consider their skin tone. The following are the 6

Fitzpatrick skin types along with their characteristics such as skin color, sun reaction, tanning abilities, and associated details.

The features listed of each Fitzpatrick type are common examples and characteristics. These characteristics are not limited to the above.

FITZPATRICK SCALE

To select a pigment mixture for your client, there are several factors to consider. These factors include, but are not limited to, skin undertone, skin tone, the color of the brow hair, the color of the client's hair, if they have previous work, and the color of their previous work.

01

SKIN UNDERTONE

The first step to pigment selection is to determine the client's undertone. Identifying whether your client has a cool, warm or neutral undertone will allow you to select the undertone of your pigments.

02

SKIN TONE

The second step to pigment selection is to determine the client's skin tone and what Fitzpatrick number they fall under. This will allow you to determine how light or how dark your pigment mixture should be.

03

FINALIZATION

Once you have determined the pigment undertone based off the client's undertone, we then select how dark the pigments should be based off of the client's skin tone. Once that has been selected, we use other factors such as the client's brow hair color, brow density, hair color, and client's preferences to finalize our pigment selection.

PIGMENT SELECTION

To select a pigment mixture for your client, there are several factors to consider. These factors include, but are not limited to, skin undertone, skin tone, the color of the brow hair, the color of the client's hair, if they have previous work, and the color of their previous work.

PIGMENT MIXTURE

PRE PROCEDURE GUIDELINES CONSULTATION

Shape

Style

Pigment

Test Patch

Medical/Skin Conditions

Client consultation to us is the most important factor to creating a good relationship with the client from the start.

During the consultation meeting, we make sure to talk about the following key terms with the client:

ALWAYS REMEMBER

During the first procedure, it is important to stay light and conservative. You can always darken during the second procedure but it's harder to make it lighter.

During the second procedure you can fine tune. If the client chooses to go thicker on the first appointment, explain that you may go thicker on the next appointment, remind them that you can never go thinner at the second appointment if they decide later that it is too thick.

DESIRE VS. NEED

Your client might want a specific color or look but it is your responsibility to guide them in the right direction for the best look. You must remember that you are the professional and that you make the ultimate decision to combine between their ultimate desire and your skills.

Consultation records:

1. medical history

2. emotional condition

3. natural skin tone

4. skin sensitivity

5. signatures

6. client expectations

7. treatment records - area treated, treatment method, color pigments used, time and duration, needle type and usage, treatment outcome.

Be over the age of 18

Not be pregnant or breastfeeding

Have obtained a doctor written consent if they are currently undergoing chemotherapy or suffer from an immune condition

Be aware that they will not be able to give blood for one year following their treatment.

Be aware that if they are to have an MRI, it should be made aware that they have permanent make up.

The continuous rapid needle penetration damages the tissue and may present itself as a sharp/scratchy pain.

Stretching the skin. While it is necessary to stretch the skin for good practice, it could cause the client some discomfort, especially as the tissue has been damaged.

The anesthetics and cleansers used are chemical irritants and can cause what some may consider to be a painful sensation, especially when used around the eyes for example.

Application of anesthetic

Scheduling appointments around the female client's monthly cycle

Working accurately and with speed

Giving necessary breaks at client's request

Use cooling antiseptic products throughout the treatment to ease discomfort

Adopting the correct stretching technique

CONSENT FORMS AND ELIGIBILITY

Your client must declare their medical history and give their signed consent to you carrying out the treatment before you begin.

They should also:

DOES IT HURT?

Remember that pain is experienced at differing levels with each individual client and that it is felt because of causing damage to the tissues of the body. During the permanent cosmetic procedure, pain can be derived in several ways:

It is likely that your client will experience some level of pain, and while you should use anesthetics to minimize this, your client should not be deluded into thinking that this is a pain-free procedure, nor should they be made to worry that this painful sensation is abnormal. You may wish to mention to your client that she will be more sensitive during her period and that it is normal to experience pain more on one side of the body than the other because of the positioning of our nerve endings.

YOU WILL MINIMIZE THE PAIN BY PATCH TEST

Auto-immune conditions (these require doctors' consent prior to treatment) Antabuse (must be finished course of medication) Insulin dependent diabetes Epilepsy

Hemophilia

HIV/Aids

Hepatitis B and C

Pregnancy and Breastfeeding

Problems with skin healing

Roaccutane - Must allow 6 months after completing the course before having

Lupus treatment

Undergoing chemotherapy – Need doctors' consent prior to treatment

It is important to always patch test the client in advance of their treatment following manufacturers' instructionsTechnicians need to be aware of how to perform an onsite scratch test if they are required to carry one out.

As has previously been mentioned, a contraindication to micropigmentation is a condition that serves as a purpose for a person not undergoing the semi permanent make up treatment. If your client admits to having one of these conditions, you should not carry out the treatment.

This list below is not exhaustive, but these are the most common contraindications preventing a client from having treatment. You should also check with your insurance company as they may put exclusion clauses in your public and product liability insurance relating to certain conditions.

A patch test should be given to the client at least 24 hours prior to them having their treatment to help determine whether they have an allergy to either the pigment or anesthetic. If the client comes to the clinic, a small dot of pigment and anesthetic should be applied to an inconspicuous part of their body, for example behind the ear. If you are posting their patch test to them, you may wish to send a cotton bud that has some of the pigment and anesthetic on it which they can rehydrate and apply to themselves.

HAIRLINE DESIGN

The process begins after the hairline is determined and approved by the patient. One of the things we frequently encounter with our patients is one of the most important aspects of hair treatment: How can you draw the Hair Line? How Should the best hairline design by female and male be?

Creating a natural hairline by female and male has always been one of the most important elements of a successful hair treatment Where the new hairline will be drawn on the scalp differs from person to person. It is determined by facial features, size of the head, ethnicity, age, hair type, the area to be transplanted, and the original hairline the patient once had. A patient over the age of 40 will have a higher hairline because when we get older, what is normal and expected is our hairline going up. Also, people in northern Europe generally have a higher hairline than people in the Mediterranean and the Middle East.

A simple method is that the patient is asked to raise his eyebrows. Just above the forehead wrinkles gives roughly FHL. (It is 2 fingers above the raised eyebrow.)

GOLDEN RATIO

Your head must be clean, or it will not work. You must PLASTIC WRAP, or it will not work. Plastic wrap is essential. You must keep it sealed from oxygen when sitting on your head. Leave It on For a Full Hour.

Most numbing solutions on the market today that can be found in beauty stores are too weak. Hence the need for numbing cream with 11% lidocaine and other ingredients to help the lidocaine seep into your client's skin. For the numbing cream to be effective, it needs to sit on your client's head for at least 45 minutes and be covered in a plastic wrap to trap the moisture in. It must be applied in a thick layer, dabbed on. At least 1/8th inch of thickness covering the entire area to be worked on. It will last about 1 to 2 hours after that, which is why you need to numb the head in sections as you work on it.

If your client tells you ahead of time they want to be numbed, you can give them an individual numbing bottle and hand them the instructions that will come with these one-time use bottles.

NUMBING

When they come in, you will remove the plastic wrap from the section that they wrapped up with the numbing cream and then apply the numbing cream on the next section of the head. You will continue moving down the head in sections. You will want to divide the head up into 4 or 5 sections depending on how long it will take to get through. Each section should take an hour.

If your client realized that they want numbing after you've already begun the procedure, you can start numbing the next section you're going to work on and either continue through the pain of the current section or cover the current section as well and just wait it out 45 minutes. After they're numb, you would continue down the head in sections as previously mentioned.

Note: Be sure to wipe away the numbing cream COMPLETELY before you begin performing SMP on the individual. If you do not wipe away all numbing cream, it can mix with the pigment when entering the skin and can result in the pigment not staying in the skin. Draw out the area you will be working on prior to beginning the treatment.

DRAW

Ideal follicle cluster pattern

Practice with a pen or pencil

The more dense your clients hair the more close together these follicle clusters should be.

DRAW ON THE HAIRLINE

FILL IN THE FRONT INCH OF THE HAIRLINE WITH THE SMP 1 NEEDLES. FILL THE

TEMPLES WITH SMP 1 OR SMP 2 NEEDLES.

FILL IN THE REST OF THE HEAD USING NEEDLES RECOMMENDED IN THE COLOR

TOOLS & SUPPLIES

Bed (Massage/Beauty Bed)

Stool

Work tray

Light (Ring light, Glamcor, etc.)

Mirror (Handheld and/or wall mirror)

Sink

Trash

Sharps container

Procedural Items

SMP Certified Machine

SMP Certified Power Source

4 x SMP Certified Needles

1 x SMC Charcoal Black Ink

1 x SMC Medium Black Ink

1 x SMC Soft Black Ink

1 x Depth Practice Sheet

4 x Ink Wells

1 x Mannequin Head

12 x Headline Stencils

2 x Synthetic Practice Skin

4 x Disposable Grips

CHECKLIST YOU WILL NEED IN YOUR SMP TRAINING KIT

WORKSPACE

DETERMINING PIGMENT AND NEEDLE SIZE TO USE FOR SMP

WHY IS THE SAME PIGMENT USED FOR DIFFERENT HAIR COLORS?

When hair is grown out (long), you can see the various subtle colors of the hair shafts. There are hundreds of different distinct hair colors. However, when hair is shaved down short, this variety of hair color does not exist. Light is no longer shining through the hair, giving it its distinct color properties. At these short lengths, the noticeable color change in hair is very slight. With the client's skin color playing a much greater role in determining which pigment to use at this hair length, only the 3 color distinctions are necessary. Same can be said when you are filling in a client's thinning hair. When filling in thinning hair, you are simply creating a shadowy cast of the hair, not their exact hair color. Example, if a blonde person has thinning hair, adding a light yellow/blonde color to their scalp with do nothing for them, except cause a lot of pain and wasted time.

The whole point, with thinning hair, is to hide the scalp by making it darker.

HOW DO I KNOW WHICH NEEDLE SIZE TO USE?

You'll notice, on each needle size recommendation in the color chart, you are given 2 different options regarding what size to use. As you become more familiar with how each needle size looks in the skin, it is best to start on the safe side, and always go with the smaller of the recommended needle sizes. As you gain more experience, regarding client's age/skin tone/ hair thickness, you will be able to more easily determine when to use which size.

HOW DO I PROPERLY WORK ON GRAY HAIR?

When someone has gone completely gray/white, and they are bald, they must shave their hair all the way down. At this time, you would need to cover their entire head (around the ears and down the back of their head). Create a lighter density by spacing the follicle points out to create a graying (salt and pepper) look.

DOES THE COLOR CHART APPLY TO SCARS AS WELL?

Yes, but most scars will require an SMP2 or SMP3 needle as scar skin is thicker and pushes pigment out easily.

DOES THE COLOR CHART APPLY TO FILL-INS ON THINNING HAIR?

Yes, the color chart applies to thinning hair as well. Please see the answer under " Why is the same pigment used for different hair colors?" section above.

PROTOCOLS & TECHNIQUES SET UP

Wash your hands with warm water & liquid soap for at least 20-30 seconds. Put on disposable gloves. Sanitize your work area with your medical-grade wipes (bed, stool, tray, ring light, etc.)

Replace your disposable gloves with a new set of gloves and put on your PPE (apron, masks, etc.) Set up your work bed and chair. First wipe down your work bed with Cavi Wipes or your chosen medical-grade cleaning supply. Put on a disposable bed sheet over the entire bed and the dental chair cover to cover the top of the bed where the client's head rest. Put a dental chair cover over your stool.

Set up your ring light. Wipe down your ring light and apply single-use barrier film on top of the areas you will touching during the procedure. Set up your work tray by covering the tray with a dental chair cover and a dental bib.

SETUP

The following are steps to properly set up your workstation:

01

Take off and dispose your soiled gloves. Wash your hands and put on a brand-new set of gloves.

02

Remove the sharps from your workstation (needles & razor blade) and dispose them into a sharps container.

03

Remove any barrier film/clip cord sleeve/grip tape from your PMU machine. Set aside the machine for cleaning.

04

Remove any barrier film and plastic cover from your workstation (bed, chair & ring light). Toss them onto your workstation tray and lift the dental chair cover. This acts as a trash bag, so we don't have to toss away any trash individually. Throw this into a hazardous waste trash

05

Sanitize your workstation by wiping any surfaces you touched or equipment you used. This includes, but is not limited to, bed, work tray, stool (and stool handle), ring light, PMU machine, etc.

BREAKDOWN

Client will need to remove piercings if obstructing treatment site area

The client should be positioned at the head of the treatment couch ensuring you have good access to the procedure area Completed and understood all the pre-procedure documentation?

Followed the pre-procedure advice and understands the importance of following post-procedure advice?

Agreed to the design and color planned for the treatment?

Agreed to pre- and post-photographs?

CLIENT PREPARATION

Following the consultation and full explanation of the treatment procedure the client should be instructed with the following guidelines before treatment commences:

CREATING COLOR

When choosing your colors, you should bear in mind that initially following an enhancement, the area will look 40% darker than the expected true pigment color following healing (4 weeks post procedure). During the follow up visit the color can be checked and any adjustments can be made to ensure client satisfaction. It really is a '2 treatment process', and your client should be made aware that the color will not be the final color after only one procedure.

THE PROCEDURE

You must consider that even though a contraindication check has taken place, a client may not always be aware if they are suffering from a general skin infection or medical condition. As a SMP artist, you should be checking the scalp area for any noticeable contraindications as well as looking at the skin type, hair type and condition. It is imperative that all hygiene practices are implemented to minimize the risk of cross infection. Before you begin, has the client?

DENSITY WILL DETERMINE HOW DARK THE SCALP WILL BE.

For people with thicker/darker side hair, you will want to make their follicle points closer together. For thinner hair, or salt and pepper hair, you will want to space the points out more to create a lighter impression. Below is an example of two extremes that help to illustrate this point. Blending is the process of creating a seamless transition from the real hair to the treated area. All SMP treatments require a degree of blending. It is without doubt a highly skilled process and perhaps the most challenging task facing your practitioner. All HIS Hair

HOW EXACTLY DOES IT WORK, AND WHAT ARE THE OPTIONS?

Depending on the extent of your hair loss, blending takes place in different parts of your scalp. If you have lost most of your hair and are (for example) at Norwood 7 level (see Norwood Hamilton Scale for more information), the blending area is where your 'horseshoe' meets your balding upper scalp. For diffuse thinners, blending takes place across your entire upper scalp and for those with advanced (Norwood 4-5) hair loss, blended areas will be wherever your remaining hair meets areas without hair.

Blending pigment dots with real hair is achieved by using a scattered gradient pattern into the real hair. The borders of the real hair are usually sparser, eventually reaching full density the further away from your balding areas you progress. You will use careful placement of pigmentation to blend a gradient of dots with the gradient of the natural hair to achieve a seamless transition. An extremely high level of skill is required to achieve optimal results.

The photograph above was taken immediately after a treatment session. You can clearly see the gradient pattern of blending used to ensure that when the dots shrink and fade, a perfect blend is achieved.

There are two primary factors that most influence how the treatment is blended – the density of your remaining hair, and the look you aim to achieve.

BLENDING

THE OPTIONS

The density of the real hair is important, because to create the most seamless treatment you will usually match that with replicated hair. It is possible for you to be sparser than the real hair, an option that is particularly relevant for older clients who want an age-appropriate look, but to go for higher density than the real hair at the back and sides is not usually appropriate.

There are exceptions of course. If the natural hair density is very sparse, you may wish to bulk it up, however this will most likely require additional pigments to be added to the back and sides to artificially increase the density of the real hair too. This way, a seamless blend can be achieved with increased density across the entire scalp.

If you have a hair transplant scar to conceal, increasing your overall density may be an appropriate option because the higher the density, the easier it is to achieve a full camouflage of your scar. Hair transplant surgery may have compromised the 'natural' density too, so this could be a good approach in some cases.

The look you aim to achieve is also important. Older clients, particularly those who have lost a lot of hair, may not desire a fully dense treatment because the change could be deemed too dramatic. A sparser look is likely to raise less questions from those around them because the change is less pronounced.

Finally, they may choose not to have a typical seamless blend, but rather, have darker pigmentation on the upper scalp than at the back and sides. Why would a client choose to do this? It's an increasingly common request made by our clients, especially among those with particularly fair hair, or with men of Afro Caribbean or African American ethnicity who can get away with very dark pigments due to the darker color of their skin. The resulting appearance is of a 'fade' style, and it looks extremely natural when executed correctly.

CREATING A NATURAL HAIRLINE THROUGH SMP

Find the sweet spot on the forehead. The rule of thumb is to measure four horizontal fingers from the area between the eyebrows to the forehead and that spot is the lower limit of the hairline, but in fact, a natural hairline should be above this point. Clients over the age of 35 usually want a less defined line, so there will be some feathering involved when creating the hairline. Feathering creates a gradient effect in which the SMP follicles gradually increase in density from the edge of the hairline toward the crown. This effect is key because natural hairlines are structured in this way. The farther back you move from the forehead, the closer the hair follicles are to one another.

A defined hairline gives a more youthful look and works well on some people.

Using two to three different shades of pigment. This technique requires considerable skill. A lighter pigment is used towards the front of the hairline and darker ones towards the back of the head. After the treatments as the pigment begins to fade, the benefits of using different shades becomes apparent.

FEATHER THE FEATHER!

Feathering the hairline is the most difficult part of creating a natural hairline. It not only takes a trained eye to scatter the

SMP dots precisely, but varying degrees of pressure must be applied to maximize the effect. The results are not only a feathering of scattered dots, but a feathering of scattered dots that are of varying shades and sizes. Not all follicles are created equal.

It takes multiple sessions. Everyone's skin is different. Some have oily skin. Some have drier skin. Some have thicker skin. Some have thinner skin. Some have lighter skin. Some have darker skin. There is no way to know how a client's skin will react to the pigment. I've had clients that retained 90 percent of the pigment, while some only retain 25 percent. The use of high-quality pigments, client's adherence to after-care instructions, and the artist's ability to be patient and know how to compensate for the lightening of the pigment all play crucial roles in the results. Therefore, we spread out SMP treatments over the course of two-to four sessions. It's a proven method that guarantees amazing results. There are many shops who claim to be able to complete your SMP treatment in one-session. A word of advice for those considering a one-treatment shop: run and don't look back!

Work with your client for the best results. After session one of their SMP treatment, the client will have a week or so to live with their new look. Most likely when they return for session two or three, they will request some modifications.

As a SMP professional you should know that if you initially go too dark, you cannot go lighter, as well as if you go too low, you cannot raise the hairline after. If the hairline you create is too well defined and low on the forehead, it may be difficult to feather it for a more gradual flow because the technique requires that you go even lower on the forehead.

Sometimes a client will want a lower hairline than should be done in the first session. It is your job to educate them about the procedure and make recommendations.

PROCEDURE

When using the pigments, pen, and/or needles for the purpose of scalp micropigmentation, stay within the following guidelines for best results and business practice:

1. Agree on price. We generally stay within the guidelines of $50 per square inch of coverage in completely bald areas, but your prices may be lower in the beginning of your business until you gain more experience.

2. Draw out the desired hairline ahead of time.

3. Clean scalp thoroughly (Scalp Wipes).

4. If using a tattoo power supply, make sure the frequency is set to 11 volts and the pedal is plugged into the left input and the pen is plugged into the right input.

5. Shake the pigment bottle well before filling your ink cap. Wipe the tip of the pigment bottle when finished so no pigment hardens and blocks the nozzle.

6. Perform a test patch to gauge client's pain tolerance. If they will be needing the numbing cream apply it to a section

of the scalp now as it will take about 45 minutes to kick in and will last about an hour. We break the head out into 4 sections for numbing, as it may take 4 hours to get through the entire head, numbing the next section as you go.

7. Remember to wipe the tip of the pigment bottle each time you use it to reduce the risk of the tip getting clogged.

8. With the pen running, adjust the needle by twisting the pen which will either extend or contract the needle. Let the needle stick out about 2mm (the small top of the needle should only enter the skin about 0.5 mm into the skin).

9. Begin pigmenting the scalp in small clusters by stepping on the power pedal with each replicated follicle being about 0.5mm to 1mm apart depending on how dense the client's existing hair is. Cluster them closer together if you are trying to achieve greater density (darker look) and more spaced out for less density(a lighter look). If you're right-handed, start working from a left to right approach so as not to smudge your work.

10.Your needle should not go deeper than 1 mm into the skin. Try to keep the needle at about 0.5 to 0.75 mm deep into the skin for each follicle.

11.Each follicle point should be just a little touch on the surface of the scalp lasting a half of a second (see videos of this procedure being performed).

12. Always be spreading the skin with your other hand so you have a taut canvas to work on.

13. For most clients, starting with SMP-1 needles along the front inch of the hairline is recommended, and then use your color chart to determine which needle size to use throughout the rest of the head.

14. You can wait to wipe off excess pigment on the scalp until after you have completed a section. Make sure your pigmented follicles show, if you see nothing but a tiny red speck, you need to go into that spot again as it did not take.

15. Use anti-redness liquid to temporarily reduce the redness and allow your client to see the results immediately.

16. Wait 1 week between sessions (or 5 to 10 days). 2 to 3 sessions are typically required.

17. 1 full top of scalp should take you about 3 - 5 hours per session depending on the size of the head and your skill level.

18. Your client should apply an ointment such as Aquaphor in between sessions.

FIRST SESSION

Before: you will be answering questions, agreeing on price, and drawing out the hairline.

During: Using the SMP-1 needle, follow along the front hairline that you drew keeping the follicle point spaced out in no order in the first half inch. Everything behind that can be part of your standard pattern that you will be doing throughout the rest of the head. See the color chart to see which needle size to use.

This technique of spacing the dots out as you approach the front hairline should be applied throughout the edges of baldness as you fade into the natural end of hair loss along the back and sides.

After: Wiping the pigment away will reveal dots that you may have missed, or areas that look too sparse and you want to fill them in more. There will be redness when you wipe all excess pigment away. You can use the Redness Remover at this point so your client can see what it will look like. Once they've had a look at it, go ahead and wipe some ointment (Aquaphor or ointment) on their head, give them the aftercare instructions and schedule the second session.

SECOND SESSION

Before: You will notice some of the points did not stay. This is due to variations in the skin and how it heals, and it may also be due to inconsistencies in your technique. You will get better and better at this over time. Explain to the client that the overall look will get darker and darker with each session. This session should take about the same amount of time as the first.

During: While filling in areas that are completely gone, you are also going to fill in areas that are just a little lighter, but still visible. It is ok to go right back into a fading follicle point as it would have disappeared with another week of healing anyway.

After: It will be a little less red this time. Same ointment procedure/aftercare instructions apply to the second session as they did on the first session.

THIRD SESSION

Before: You will see a lot less fading, if any, on this session. There will be minimal work to do, so just look all around the head and decide which areas you are going to work on.

During: You should look at the client's head up closely, and then look at it from a distance (about 2-3 feet back) to get a full picture of what areas need any touching up.

After: Even less redness will be present as less work has been done. The client should continue putting ointment on their head for the next 7 days and follow the aftercare instructions.

The most common form of scar work being done with scalp micropigmentation is the camouflaging of hair transplant scars. To properly camouflage a hair transplant scar, you must first understand what they are and how they are created. First, you must first understand that hair naturally gets thinner as it goes down the back of your head.

When a traditional strip-scar hair transplant is done, a large strip of the scalp, from ear to ear, is removed from the back of the client's head. This makes the thicker hair press up against the thinner hair, which doesn't look right. It no longer has the natural fade that existed prior to the procedure. You will notice, in the image, that the thicker hair up top and the thinner hair below no longer have a natural fade from one to another.

SCAR WORK

Your goal, when working on scars, is to recreate the blending from thicker to thinner hair that was once there for your client. To do this, you must start by filling in the scar itself, using SMP-3 needles, then work your way down (below the scar) and space out your follicles more and more as you go down. You should go down about 1 or 2 inches Doing this recreates the fading effect of a natural hairline along the back of the head down to the neck.

BLENDING

When blending into the client's hair throughout the sides and back of their head, it is important to NOT come to a hard stopping point. You should space out the follicle points as you start to run into the existing hair so that the transition is smooth and undetectable.

In this example, we will show the blending into longer hair, so the distinction is apparent.

REDNESS REMOVER INSTRUCTIONS

Directions for using the Redness Remover After performing scalp micropigmentation, SMP, your client's head will be red because of the procedure. This unique formula helps reduce the redness of the client's head and allows them to see the results of the SMP procedure immediately. After spraying the client's scalp with the Redness Remover, wait 2 to 3 minutes to see the redness go away. This is temporary and will last for about 15 minutes before the redness returns. Apply healing ointment such as Aquaphor, after the redness remover has taken effect.

Note: You must put it on generously and do not cover the skin with any ointment prior to doing spraying the redness remover.

SPOT REMOVER INSTRUCTIONS

If a needle point of yours goes in too deep, or you are dealing with a client that has had previous work done that they want removed, you can use Spot Remover to remove small points. If the entire head needs to have the SMP removed, you will want to advise your client to.

DIRECTIONS FOR PIGMENT/BAD SMP REMOVAL

The needle should be set to go no deeper than 1.5 mm. Use an SMP-5 needle. Poor the Spot Remover in a small sterile ink cup. Dip the needle into Spot Remover. Go into the smp follicle point itself in a circular motion. No more than four passes should be made. Only use removal on area no larger than a 2 mm diameter. The area should be bleeding slightly if this was done correctly. It can take up to 2 to 3 procedures 30 days apart to see the tattooed/pigmented area lightened or removed. Skin condition and the deepness of a tattoo will also be a determining factor if the tattoo is able to be removed or lightened.

WHAT ARE THE AFTERCARE INSTRUCTIONS?

Directly after the procedure is complete disinfect with Isopropyl Alcohol. Customer should remain still for 5-10 minutes and let the blood coagulate and start the scab. Advise client to keep the area dry for 24 hours to form a scab. When washing or showering, only wash gently with fingers and pat dry. Never soak in water. No creams or any kind of makeup. The scab is the tool to remove the pigment and should not be picked. Let scab fall off naturally. After the scab is gone and completely healed, rub vitamin E into the skin once daily and do not repeat the procedure for a minimum of four weeks.

The spot remover is tattooed into the dermis containing unwanted color (pigment); microscopic scar tissue containing the pigment in the dermis slightly rises for approximately 12 hours, the dermis layer of the skin forms a scab and adheres to the pigment particles. Once the scab falls off, either most or some of the pigment will leave the body. There is no way to predict the number of sessions needed due to the different depths the pigment is inserted and types of pigment.

For instant removal of SMP work:

1. For large areas, laser removal may be necessary. Recommend your client to a professional in your area.

2. For smaller areas or individual points, skin tone pigments can be used to cover up the smp ink/pigment. There are plenty of skin tone pigments on the market, but we recommend Complexion Correction as it does not bleed/blend into the existing points. It covers them instantly and it allows you to mix the pigment to match the clients exact skin color, effectively making the client's smp disappear immediately.

AFTERCARE

Sweating heavily – Try not to engage in any intense exercise for 5 days following treatment. Excessive sweating could interrupt the healing process Scrubbing and shampooing –

Scrubbing the scalp can break the skin and open wounds, and shampooing could introduce harsh chemicals.

Shaving – Avoid shaving and irritating the area while it's healing. Exposure to long-term sunlight – UV rays from the sun can cause sunburn and sun damage. This could lead to premature fading of the scalp pigmentation.

Touching with hands – Refrain from touching your scalp with your hands too much. You could introduce bacteria and increase the risk of infection.

Scalp micropigmentation involves using tiny microneedles to deposit pigment into the shallow skin layers of the scalp. During the healing process, new skin layers will grow over where the pigment was placed. Once the scalp is completely healed, you'll be left with scalp micropigmentation that looks natural and undetectable. After your treatment session, it's important that you're following a routine for scalp micropigmentation aftercare.

AFTERCARE TIPS IN THE DAYS FOLLOWING YOUR SESSION

In general, you'll want to treat your scalp like an open wound after SMP treatment. Meaning, avoid getting it wet and keep it clean. No chlorinated pools, saunas, steam rooms, or tanning beds for 28 days after your final treatment. This will ensure a good, long-lasting result.

DAY 0 TO DAY 5

For the first 5 days following treatment, you should avoid the following:

During the first 5 days, make sure you're drinking plenty of water and taking any medication as prescribed. You can lightly rinse the scalp while it's healing and dab the area with a wet cloth to keep it clean. Do not soak the scalp. You may also wear a hat or skullcap and sleep any way that's comfortable for you.

Scratching the scalp – As with tattoos, the skin on your scalp may begin to peel during these next few days. It's important that you avoid scratching or picking any scabs that may form.

Shampooing or exfoliating – Shampoo and exfoliants can disrupt the formation of new skin layers during healing.

Using self-tanners or skin irritants – While your scalp is healing, avoid irritants that could cause inflammation and disturb the healing process.

DAY 5 TO DAY 10

For day 5 to 10, your head should be looking much better and healing nicely. However, it is still healing. You'll want to make sure you're keeping up with an aftercare routine.

For the next 5 days, you should still avoid the following:

What you can do is carefully shave or cut your hair if needed. You should also continue rinsing lightly with water and soap to clean the area. Applying a moisturizer will also help the healing stage during this time. Just make sure it's fragrance free. You can also resume working out with light exercise.

DAY 10 AND ONWARD

After 10 days, your scalp should be healed enough to return to your normal routine. You may be scheduled for your next treatment session after 10 days.

However, your next treatment date will depend on how it has healed so far. Before your next follow-up session, you'll be requested to wash your head and cut your hair.

CONCLUSIONS

Scalp micropigmentation, also known as a hair tattoo or medical hairline tattoo, is a revolutionary solution for individuals experiencing hair loss or thinning. This non-surgical, minimally invasive procedure has gained immense popularity in recent years, offering a natural-looking and long-lasting alternative to traditional hair restoration methods.

The concluding words on scalp micropigmentation highlight the transformative power of this innovative technique and its ability to restore confidence and self-esteem for those affected by hair loss.

The process of scalp micropigmentation involves using specialized techniques and pigments to create the illusion of natural-looking hair follicles on the scalp. Skilled technicians meticulously implant pigments into the scalp's dermis layer, mimicking the appearance of real hair follicles. This technique can be used to create the illusion of a fuller head of hair, restore a receding hairline, or camouflage thinning areas.

One of the significant advantages of scalp micropigmentation is its versatility. It can be tailored to suit individuals with varying degrees of hair loss, from mild thinning to complete baldness. The procedure can also be combined with other hair restoration techniques, such as hair transplants or camouflage products, for a comprehensive and personalized solution.

For individuals who have experienced the emotional toll of hair loss, scalp micropigmentation offers a transformative journey. The procedure can restore self-confidence and a sense of youthfulness, allowing individuals to embrace their appearance without the constant worry and self-consciousness associated with hair loss.

Moreover, scalp micropigmentation is a low-maintenance solution compared to other hair restoration methods. Once the procedure is complete, individuals can enjoy a natural-looking appearance without the need for daily styling or the use of hair concealers. The pigments used in the procedure are designed to be long-lasting, with touch-ups typically required every few years to maintain optimal results.

As the demand for scalp micropigmentation continues to grow, the industry is witnessing constant advancements and improvements. Highly skilled technicians undergo rigorous training to ensure precise and natural-looking results, utilizing the latest techniques and state-of-the-art pigments. Additionally, reputable clinics prioritize safety and follow strict protocols to minimize risks and ensure optimal outcomes.

In conclusion, scalp micropigmentation is a game-changer in the realm of hair restoration. Its ability to provide a natural-looking and long-lasting solution for hair loss, combined with its low-maintenance requirements and transformative effects on self-confidence, make it a compelling choice for individuals seeking a permanent and effective solution. As the industry continues to evolve, scalp micropigmentation stands as a testament to the power of innovation and the pursuit of restoring confidence and self-esteem for those affected by hair loss.

THE SMP PROGRESS KEEPER

MONTH	
YEAR	

MON	TUES	WED	THURS	SUN	FRI	SAT

TRACKER	M	T	W	TH	F	S	S

NOTES

CHANGES NOTICED

MOTIVATION

THE SMP PROGRESS KEEPER

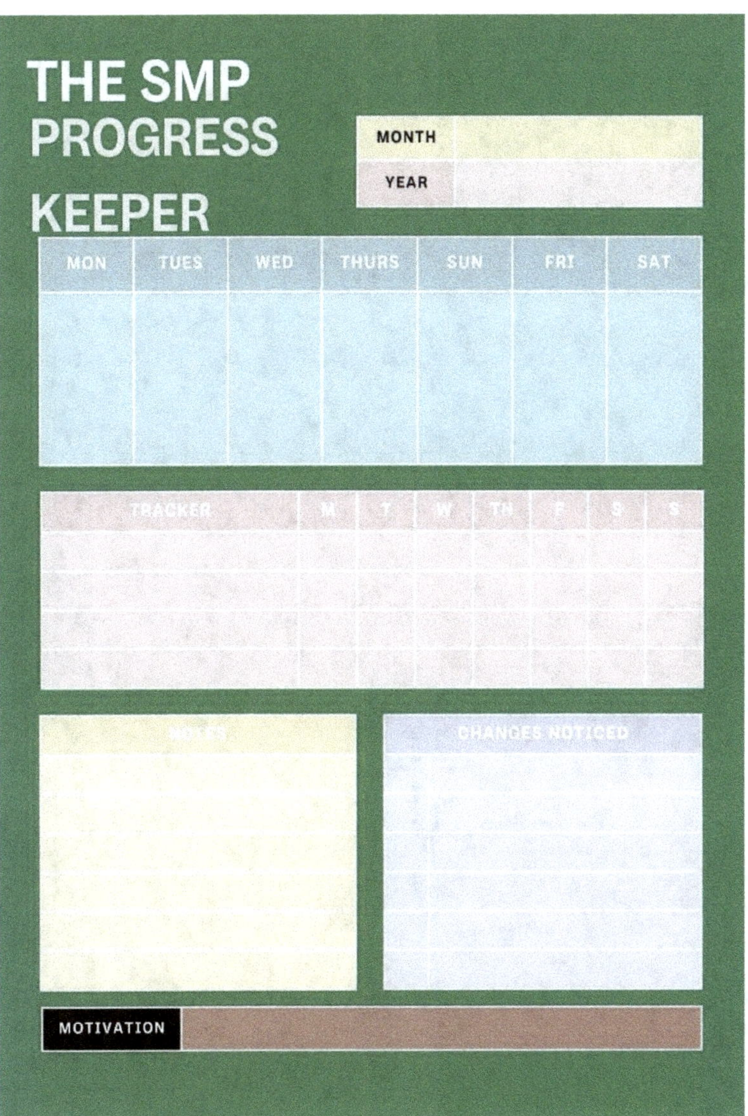

THE SMP PROGRESS KEEPER

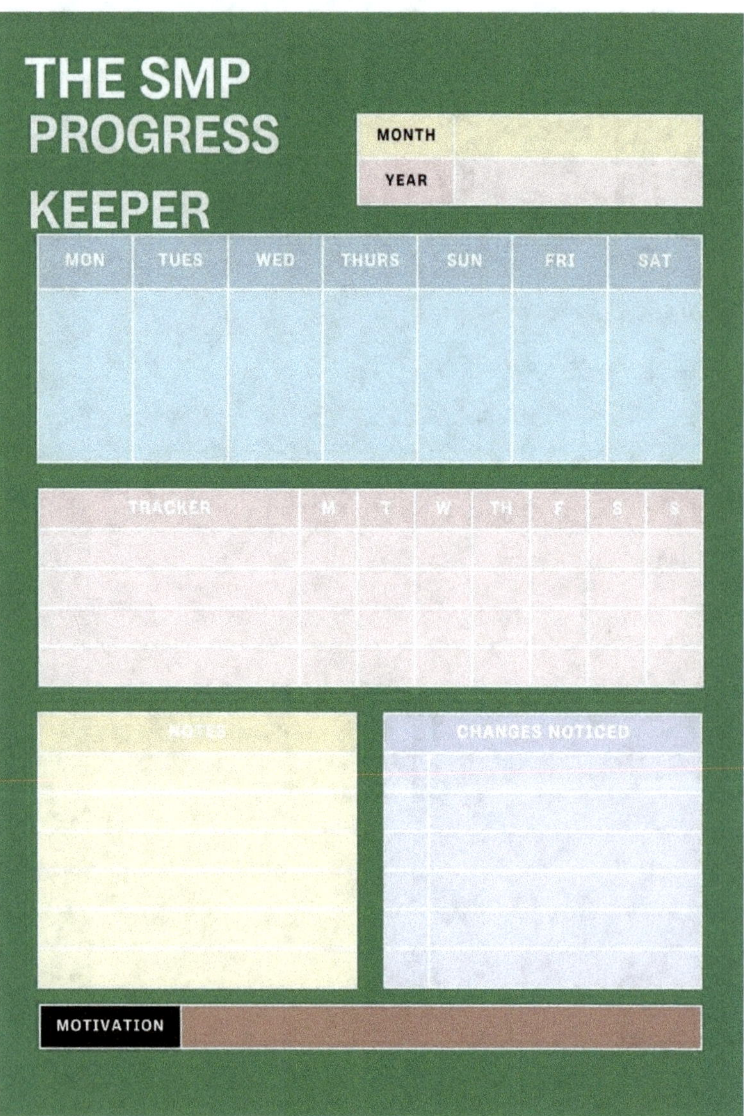

THE SMP PROGRESS KEEPER

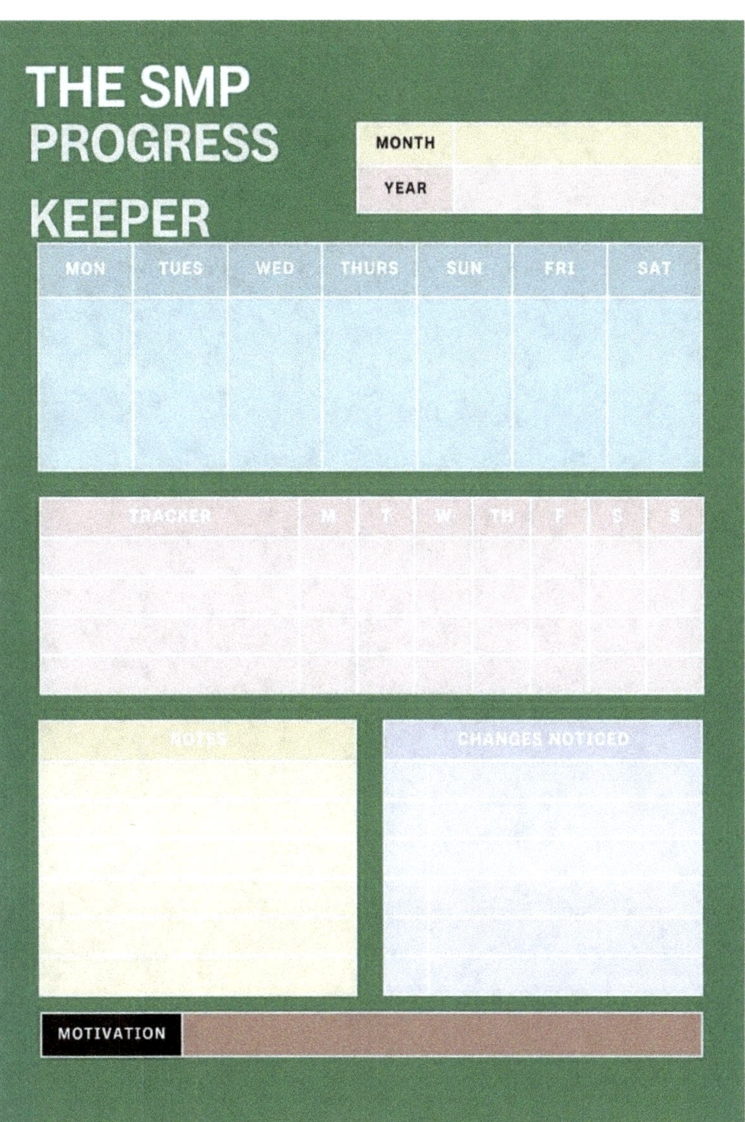